NEONATAL AND PEDIATRIC PULMONARY GRAPHICS

A Bedside Guide

Edited by

Steven M. Donn, M.D.
Professor of Pediatrics
Division of Neonatal-Perinatal Medicine
Medical Director, Holden Neonatal
Intensive Care Unit
University of Michigan Health System
Ann Arbor, Michigan

FUTURA

Futura Publishing
Company
Armonk, New York

Library of Congress Cataloging–in–Publishing Data

Neonatal and pediatric pulmonary graphics : principles and clinical applications / edited by Steven M. Donn.

    p.   cm.

Includes bibliographical references and index.

ISBN 0-87993-645-2

1. Pulmonary function tests for newborn infants. 2. Respiration—Measurement. 3. Respiratory therapy for newborn infants. I. Donn, Steven M.

[DNLM: 1. Respiratory Function Tests—in infancy & childhood 2. Ventilators, Mechanical—in infancy & childhood. 3. Monitor-ing, Physiologic—methods. 4. Respiratory System—physiology. 5. Respiratory Distress Syndrome—therapy.   WF 141 N438 1997]

RJ312.N45   1997

618.92′24075—dc21

DNLM/DLC

for Library of Congress   97-39522
                                                         CIP

Contributors

Jeanette Asselin, M.S., R.R.T.
Manager, Neonatal/Pulmonary Research
Children's Hospital of Oakland
Oakland, CA

Lindon A. Baker, B.S.E.T.E.
Principal Engineer
LAB Engineering Services
Yorba Linda, CA

Kenneth P. Bandy, R.R.T.
Technical Director
Department of Respiratory Care
University of Michigan Health System
Ann Arbor, MI

Michael A. Becker, R.R.T.
Clinical Specialist-Neonatal Intensive Care
Department of Respiratory Care
University of Michigan Health System
Ann Arbor, MI

Vinod K. Bhutani, M.D.
Professor of Pediatrics
Section on Newborn Pediatrics
Pennsylvania Hospital
Philadelphia, PA

Dennis Bing, R.R.T.
Development Leader
Infant Pulmonary Research
  Center
Children's Health Care
St. Paul, MN

M. Douglas Cunningham, M.D.
Professor of Pediatrics
University of California-Irvine
Director of Neonatology
Miller Children's Hospital
Long Beach, CA

Douglas F. DeVries, B.S.M.E.
Vice President, Engineering
Bird Products Corporation
Palm Springs, CA

Mary Dekeon, R.R.T.
Clinical Supervisor-Pediatric
  Intensive Care
Department of Respiratory Care
University of Michigan Health
  System
Ann Arbor, MI

Steven M. Donn, M.D.
Professor of Pediatrics
Division of Neonatal-Perinatal Medicine
Medical Director, Holden Neonatal Intensive Care Unit
University of Michigan Health System
Ann Arbor, MI

Margaret F. Everett, M.D.
Department of Pediatrics
St. Joseph Mercy Hospital
Ann Arbor, MI

Tilo O. Gerhardt, M.D.
Professor of Pediatrics
Division of Neonatology
University of Miami School of Medicine
Miami, FL

Mitchell Goldstein, M.D.
Assistant Clinical Professor of Pediatrics
University of California, Irvine
Director, Neonatal Pulmonary Medicine
Queen of the Valley Hospital
West Covina, CA

Cheryll K. Hagus, E.M.B.A., R.R.T.
Assistant Professor
Department of Respiratory Care
Southwest Texas State University
San Marcos, TX

Alain Harf, M.D., Ph.D.
Professor of Physiology
Service de Physiologie -Explorations
    Fonctionnelles
Centre Hospitalier Universitaire Henri Mondor
Universite Paris XII - Val de Marne
Creteil, France

Ronald B. Hirschl, M.D.
Assistant Professor
Division of Pediatric Surgery
Department of Surgery
University of Michigan Health System
Ann Arbor, MI

Pierre-Henri Jarreau, M.D., Ph.D.
Assistant Professor of Pediatrics
Service de Medecine Neonatale de Port-Royal
Centre Hospitalier Universitaire Cochin-Port-Royal
Universite Paris V - Rene Descarte
Paris, France

Damon Lawson, M.B.A., R.R.T.
Marketing Manager
Ventilation Products Division
Allied Healthcare Products, Inc.
Riverside, CA

Alan C. Letscher, R.R.T.
Infant Products Manager
Bird Products Corporation
Palm Springs, CA

Hubert Lorino, Ph.D.
Senior Research Fellow
Institut National de la Sante et de la Recherche
    Medicale
Unite de Recherche de Physiologie Respiratoire
Faculte de Medecine de Creteil
Creteil, France

Christian Mariette, B.Sc.
Computer Scientist
Service de Physiologie-Explorations Fonctionnelles
Centre Hospitalier Universitaire Henri
    Mondor
Universite Paris XII - Val deMarne.
Creteil, France

Guy Moriette, M.D.
Professor of Pediatrics
Service de Medecine Neonatale de Port-Royal
Centre Hospitalier Universitaire Cochin-Port-Royal
Universite Paris V - Rene Descartes
Paris, France

Ralph Mosca, M.D.
Assistant Professor of Surgery
Division of Pediatric Cardiothoracic Surgery
University of Michigan Health System
Ann Arbor, MI

Martha Nelson, M.D.
Clinical Instructor of Pediatrics
Division of Neonatal-Perinatal Medicine
University of Michigan Health System
Ann Arbor, MI

Joanne J. Nicks, R.R.T.
Clinical Supervisor-Neonatal Intensive Care
Department of Respiratory Care
University of Michigan Health System
Ann Arbor, MI

Paul Ouellet, R.R.T.
Manager, Respiratory Care Services
Edmundston Regional Hospital
Edmundston, New Brunswick, Canada

Tonse N. K. Raju, M.D.
Professor of Pediatrics
Division of Neonatology
University of Illinois at Chicago Medical Center
Chicago, IL

Katie Sabato, M.S., R.R.T.
Pediatric Intensive Care Unit Coordinator
Respiratory Care
Children's Hospital of Oakland
Oakland, CA

Robert E. Schumacher, M.D.
Associate Professor of Pediatrics
Division of Neonatal-Perinatal Medicine
University of Michigan Health System
Ann Arbor, MI

Sunil K. Sinha, M.D., Ph.D.
Consultant Paediatrician
Director of Neonatology
South Cleveland Hospital
Middlesbrough, United Kingdom

Emidio M. Sivieri, M.S.
Section on Newborn Pediatrics
Pennsylvania Hospital
Philadelphia, PA

Thomas A. Sondergeld, R.R.T.
Manager, Special Care Nursery
Northwestern Memorial Hospital
Chicago, IL

Wan C. Tsai, M.D.
Fellow, Pediatric Pulmonary Medicine
Department of Pediatrics
University of Michigan Health System
Ann Arbor, MI

Table of Contents

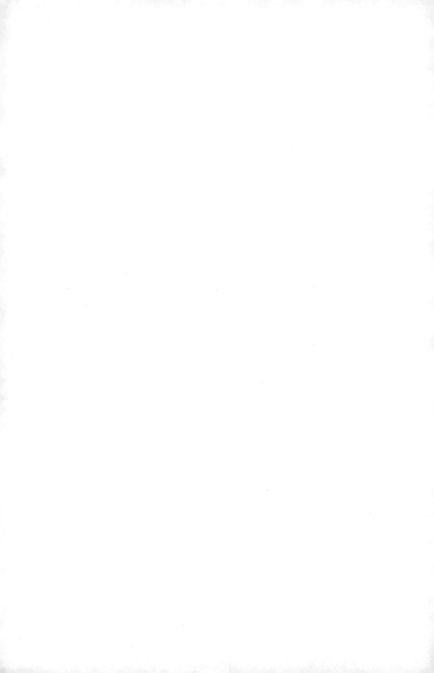

Introduction

Neonatal and Pediatric Pulmonary Graphics: A Bed-side Guide is a companion to the larger text, *Neonatal and Pediatric Pulmonary Graphics: Principles and Clinical Applications.* The examples which appear in this guide have been taken directly from the text and are presented in an abstracted form to enable the reader to have a handy reference for pulmonary waveforms and loops.

For each example, two illustrations are given. On the left-hand page is an idealized version which has been hand drawn, and which includes the major educational points of emphasis. On the right-hand page is an actual clinical representation of the same example, created by one of the commercially available devices. In each case, the specific device is identified so that the reader may become familiar with the different ways in which the various devices display data. There is also a chapter reference for a more detailed discussion of the waveform or loop depicted.

Although space precludes publication of every possible graphic example, those selected for inclusion are among the ones most commonly encountered in clinical practice.

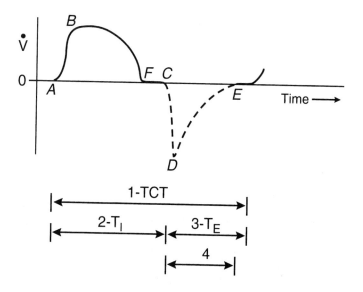

Figure: 4-2

Device: Idealized waveform

Legend: Inspiratory and expiratory flow waveform, such as that seen with time-cycled, pressure-limited mechanical ventilation. Positive deflection (above baseline) represents inspiration, whereas negative deflection (below baseline) represents expiration.

Reference: Chapters 3 and 4

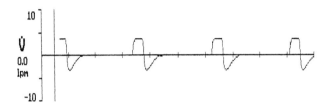

Figure: 13-4

Device: Bird Graphics Monitor

Legend: Square inspiratory flow pattern of mandatory mechanical breath, volume-controlled ventilation.

Reference: Chapter 13

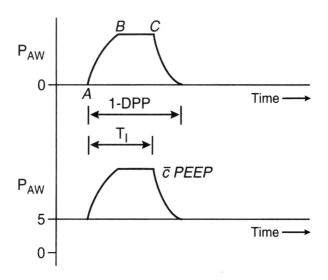

Figure: 4-6

Device: Idealized pressure waveform

Legend: Inspiratory and expiratory pressure waveform for a time-cycled, pressure-limited breath type.

Reference: Chapters 3 and 4

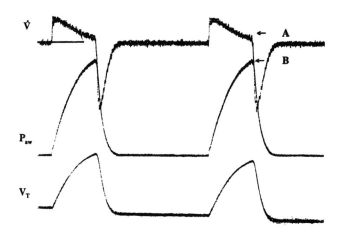

Figure: 7-5

Device: Bicore CP-100

Legend: A single breath drawing to illustrate airway pressure at points of inspiratory and expiratory flow. Note midpoint (A) equals no flow and corresponds to point B at peak airway pressure ($\dot{V}$ = flow, P_{AW} = airway pressure, and V_T = tidal volume).

Reference: Chapter 7

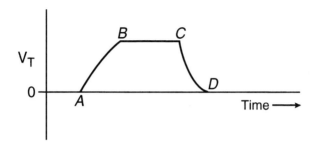

Figure: 4-8

Device: Idealized volume waveform

Legend: Inspiratory and expiratory volume waveform for a time-cycled, pressure-limited breath type.

Reference: Chapters 3 and 4

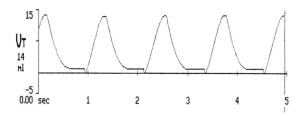

Figure: M-1 (see also 14-12)

Device: Bird Graphics Monitor

Legend: Inspiratory and expiratory volume
waveform.

Reference: Chapter 14

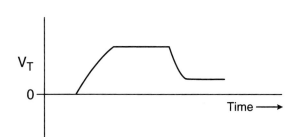

Figure: 4-9

Device: Idealized volume waveform

Legend: Inspiratory and expiratory volume waveform showing the effect of a leak in the patient circuit or around the artificial airway.

Reference: Chapter 4

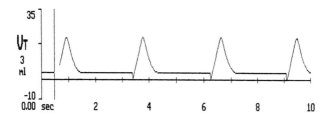

Figure: 13-12

Device: Bird Graphics Monitor

Legend: Volume waveform. Note that not all of the inspired tidal volume returns during expiration (waveform fails to reach baseline). This is suggestive of a leak.

Reference: Chapter 13

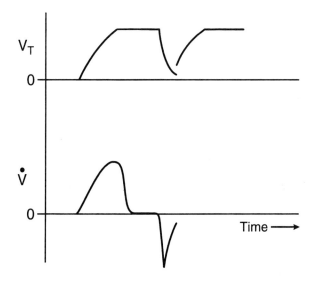

Figure: 4-10

Device: Idealized flow and volume waveforms.

Legend: Inspiratory and expiratory flow and volume waveforms showing the effect of inadequate expiratory time and the resulting air trapping.

Reference: Chapter 4

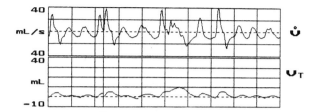

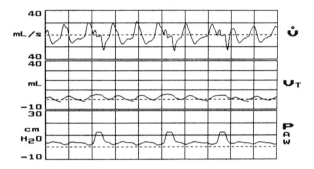

Figure: 7-14

Device: Bicore CP-100

Legend: Both of these examples of airway monitoring reveal poor synchronizing of patient and ventilator breaths. "Stacking" or superimposition of breaths is evident. Note disruption of tidal volume delivery in lower panel.

Reference: Chapter 7

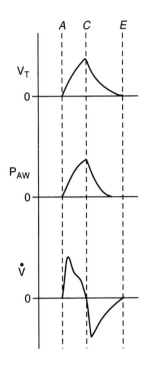

Figure: 4-12

Device: Idealized volume, pressure, and flow
waveforms

Legend: Composite volume, pressure, and flow
waveforms for a flow-triggered, pressure-limited,
flow-cycled breath type.

Reference: Chapter 4.

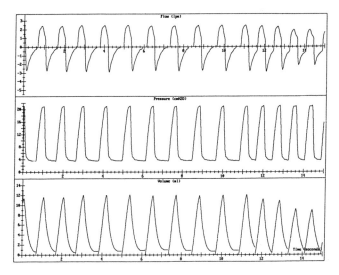

Figure: 10-6

Device: VenTrak Model 1550

Legend: VenTrak flow, pressure, and volume over time monitoring graph. Ventilator rate, by lower T_E, is increased on mechanical breaths from left to right. Expiratory gas flow does not return to baseline before the start of the next breath. Note reduced tidal volume delivery. Gas trapping is likely.

Reference: Chapter 10.

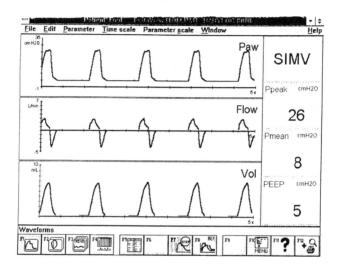

Figure: 8-3

Device: Dräger Babylog 8000

Legend: Composite pressure (P_{AW}), flow, and volume waveforms displayed in real-time during synchronized intermittent mandatory ventilation.

Reference: Chapter 8.

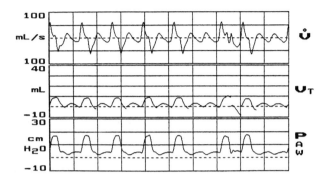

Figure: 7-8

Device: Bicore CP-100

Legend: Basic waveform displays of flow ($\dot{V}$), tidal volume (V_T), and airway pressure (P_{AW}). Note the distinctly large ventilator breaths for all three waveforms.

Reference: Chapter 7.

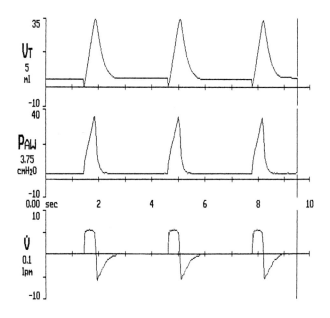

Figure: 13-19B

Device: Bird Graphics Monitor

Legend: Composite volume, pressure, and flow waveforms during volume-controlled, assist-control ventilation. Note that monitor enables user to choose two of the three waveforms for continuous real-time display.

Reference: Chapter 13.

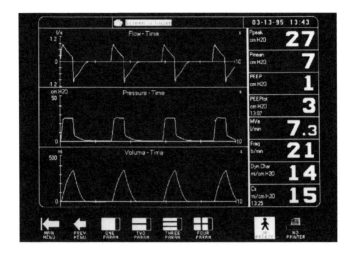

Figure: 9-4

Device: Siemens Servo Screen 390

Legend: Composite volume, pressure, and flow waveforms shown in a continuous real-time display.

Reference: Chapter 9.

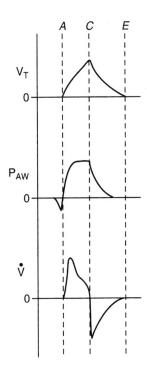

Figure: 4-21

Device: Idealized volume, pressure, and flow waveforms.

Legend: Composite volume, pressure, and flow waveforms for a spontaneous breath which is pressure-supported.

Reference: Chapters 4 and 14.

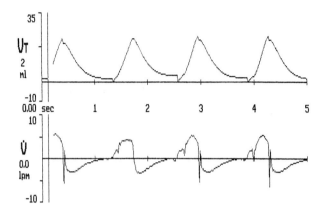

Figure: 14-1A

Device: Bird Graphics Monitor

Legend: Volume and flow waveforms during synchronized intermittent mandatory ventilation with PS_{max}. The first, third, and fourth breaths are pressure-supported and generate the same tidal volume as the second breath, which is provided by volume-controlled SIMV.

Reference: Chapter 14.

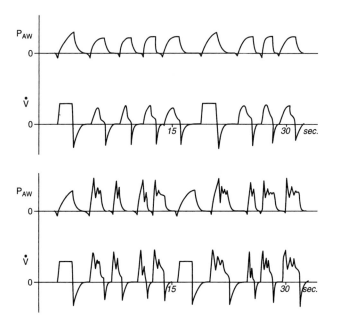

Figure: 4-27

Device: Idealized flow and pressure waveforms.

Legend: Flow and pressure waveforms showing the optimization of the pressure-support level. In the top graphic, the PS level has been titrated down resulting in the elimination of pressure overshoot and oscillation, which is depicted in the bottom graphic.

Reference: Chapter 4.

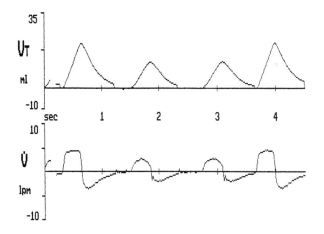

Figure: 14-1B

Device: Bird Graphics Monitor

Legend: Volume and flow waveforms during SIMV with PS. In this case, PS is used to provide partial support. Note that the second and third breaths (PS) provide a smaller tidal volume than the volume-controlled SIMV breaths (first and fourth breaths).

Reference: Chapter 14.

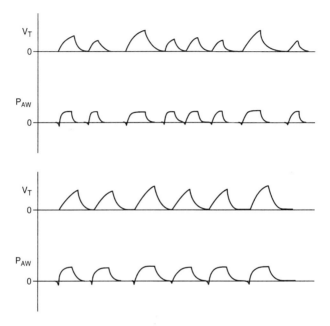

Figure: 4-28

Device: Idealized volume and pressure waveforms

Legend: Volume and pressure waveforms showing the weaning of pressure support. In the bottom
graphic, the PS level was reduced by 20% and the
respiratory rate and pattern indicate the patient is tol-
erating the wean well. In the top graphic, further reduction of the PS level results in an erratic respiratory
rate and rhythm indicating that the patient is tiring.

Reference: Chapter 4.

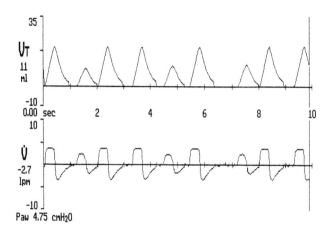

Figure: 14-4B

Device: Bird Graphics Monitor

Legend: Volume and flow waveforms during volume-controlled SIMV with PS. Note the smaller delivered tidal volume and changes in the flow waveform during the partial support provided by PS ventilation, which is largely patient controlled.

Reference: Chapter 14.

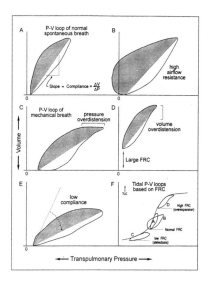

Figure: 3-5

Device: Idealized pressure-volume loops.

Legend: Characteristics of pressure-volume loops under various ventilatory conditions (A-E). The shaded area indicates the expiratory portion of the breath and the unshaded area indicates the inspiratory portion. The slope of the line connecting end-expiration to end-inspiration can be used to estimate pulmonary compliance. Panel F displays loops superimposed on the total respiratory pressure-volume relationship. The characteristics of the pressure-volume loop change as ventilation occurs along various portions of the static pressure-volume relationship.

Reference: Chapter 3.

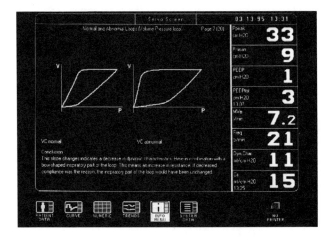

Figure: 9-9

Device: Siemens Servo Screen 390

Legend: Pressure-volume relationship displayed in real-time. Loop on left is normal, while that on the right is abnormal and represents overdistention.

Reference: Chapter 9.

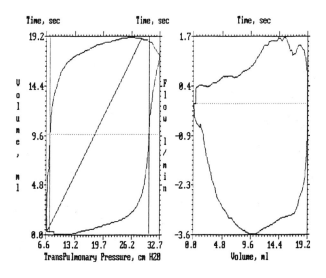

Figure: 16-4

Device: StarCalc

Legend: Pressure-volume and flow-volume loops obtained from an infant with a double aortic arch with very limited expiratory flow and decreased pulmonary compliance.

Reference: Chapter 16.

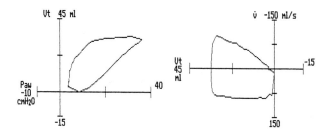

Figure: 13-17A

Device: Bird Graphics Monitor

Legend: Pressure-volume and flow-volume loops obtained from an infant with overly compliant lungs who demonstrates a vertical shift in the pressure-volume loop and overdistention of the lungs.

Reference: Chapter 13.

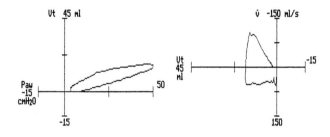

Figure: 13-17B

Device: Bird Graphics Monitor

Legend: Pressure-volume and flow-volume loops obtained from an infant with poorly compliant lungs who demonstrates a horizontal shift in the pressure-volume loop.

Reference: Chapter 13.

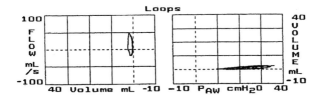

Figure: 15-9

Device: Bicore CP-100

Legend: Flow-volume and pressure-volume loops obtained from a patient with ARDS who demonstrates a horizontal shift in the pressure-volume loop indicative of extremely poor pulmonary compliance.

Reference: Chapter 15.

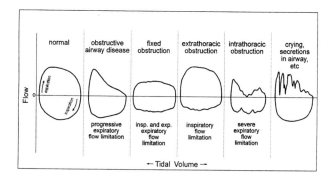

Figure: 3-7

Device: Idealized flow-volume loops

Legend: Examples of flow-volume loops under normal and various abnormal conditions.
          Note that in the actual examples which follow, the loops are not drawn in an accepted conventional manner but according to each manufacturer's preference. Users should become familiar with this variance.

Reference: Chapter 3.

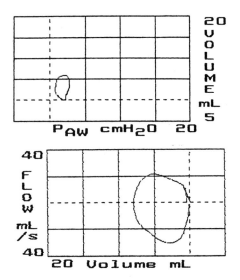

Figure: 7-17

Device: Bicore CP-100

Legend: Normal patient-generated pressure-volume loop (top) and flow-volume loop (bottom). Loops are inscribed as hysteresis between volume change and airway flow or airway pressure change.

Reference: Chapter 7.

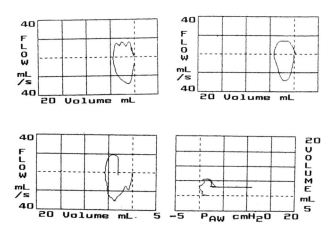

Figure: 7-21A

Device: Bicore CP-100

Legend: Flow-volume loops that give evidence for airway obstruction on expiration. Upper left suggests partial obstruction of endotracheal tube. Lower left is more suggestive of a faulty ventilator expiratory valve.

Reference: Chapter 7.

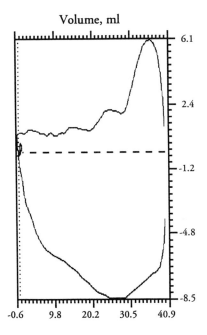

Volume, ml

Figure: 16-1

Device: StarCalc

Legend: Flow-volume loop obtained from an infant with a double aortic arch demonstrating a "fixed" airway obstruction.

Reference: Chapter 16.

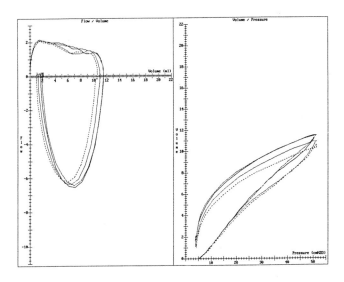

Figure: 10-4

Device: VenTrak Model 1550

Legend: Flow-volume (V̇-V) and pressure-volume (P-V) loops during IMV in an infant. Inspiration is on the positive flow -volume loop scale. A reduction in slope during the later portion of inspiration on the P-V loop demonstrates some degree of lung overdistention. A small endotracheal tube leak prevents closure on expiration.

Reference: Chapter 10.

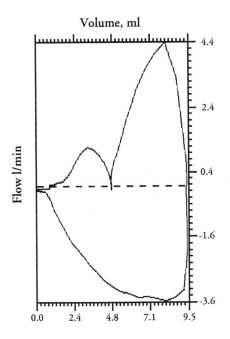

Figure: 16-2

Device: StarCalc

Legend: Flow-volume loop obtained from an infant with tracheal malacia demonstrating "dynamic" airway collapse.

Reference: Chapter 16.

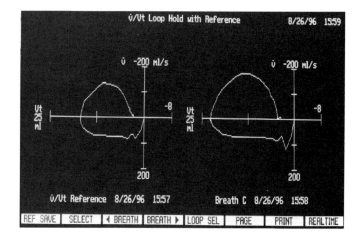

Figure: 6-7

Device: Bird Graphics Monitor

Legend: Actual screen display of two flow-volume loops taken before (left) and after (right) administration of bronchodilator therapy. Note improvement in the shape of the loop, indicating decreased resistance and increased flow.

Reference: Chapter 6.

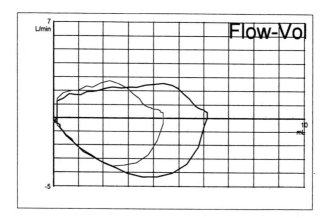

Figure: 8-6

Device: Dräger Babylog 8000

Legend: Two flow-volume loops are depicted; the reference loop (prior to administration of bronchodilator therapy) is the lighter of the two. Note improvement in the shape of the darker subsequent loop, indicating decreased resistance and increased flow.

Reference: Chapter 8.

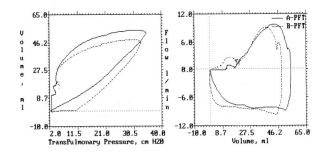

Figure: 16-12

Device: StarCalc

Legend: Pressure-volume and flow-volume
loops done in a patient positioned supine (PFT A) and
prone (PFT B). Patient has Tetralogy of Fallot and ab-
sent pulmonary valve. Note improvement in lung me-
chanics with just a change in the infant's position.

Reference: Chapter 16.

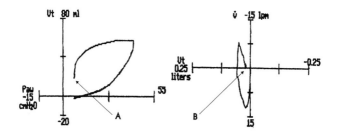

Figure: 15-2

Device: Bicore CP-100

Legend: Pressure-volume and flow-volume loops from a patient with an uncuffed endotracheal tube and a large audible air leak. Volumes indicated in A and B do not return to baseline.

Reference: Chapter 15.

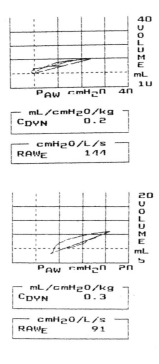

Figure: 7-23

Device: Bicore CP-100

Legend: Pressure-volume loops reflecting pre-
and post-treatment with surfactant in preterm infant
with severe respiratory distress syndrome. Note
slight improvement of compliance and decreased airway resistance.

Reference: Chapter 7.

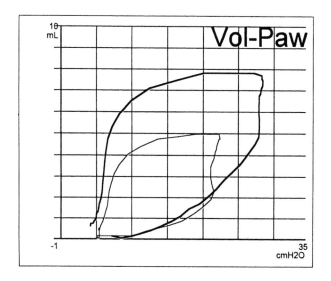

Figure: 8-5

Device: Dräger Babylog 8000

Legend: Pressure-volume loops reflecting pre- and post-treatment with surfactant in preterm infant with respiratory distress syndrome. Note improvement of compliance and decreased airway resistance. The reference loop (prior to surfactant administration) is the lighter of the two.

Reference: Chapter 8.

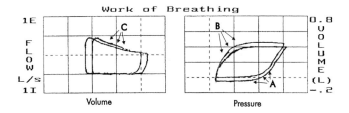

Figure: 15-12

Device: Bicore CP-100

Legend: Flow-volume and pressure-volume loops of an asthmatic patient. Note marked resistance to flow on inspiration (A) and exhalation (B), and prolonged exhalation (C).

Reference: Chapter 15.

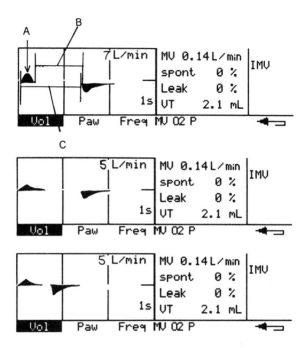

Figure: 8-2

Device: Dräger Babylog 8000

Legend: Integrated flow waveform graphics
screen demonstrating varying effects when (A) inspiratory flow is set at 7 L/min; (B) inspiratory flow is
adjusted to 5 L/min; and (C) inspiratory flow remains
at 5 L/min but inspiratory time is decreased.

Reference: Chapter 8.

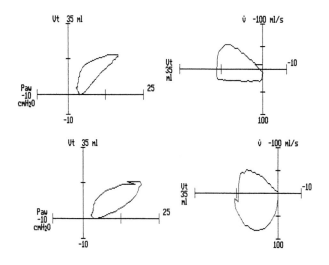

Figure: 14-5A and 14-5B

Device: Bird Graphic Monitor

Legend: Pressure-volume and flow-volume loops during volume-controlled SIMV of a patient with bronchopulmonary dysplasia (left). This infant has significantly elevated airway resistance, which results in a flattening of the inspiratory limb of the flow volume loop. Pressure-volume and flow-volume loops during straight pressure-support ventilation are shown on the right,, The variable inspiratory flow available during pressure-support ventilation enables the patient to overcome the elevated resistance. Note the now normal ovoid shape of the flow-volume loop.

Reference: Chapter 14.

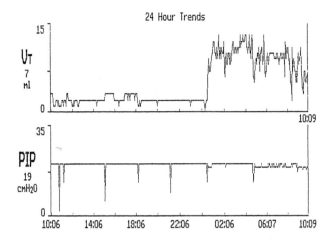

24 Hour Trends

Figure: 17-5

Device: Bird Graphic Monitor

Legend: Trend recording of tidal volume and airway pressures over a 24-hour period in an infant with meconium aspiration syndrome (who is on extracorporeal life support). There is a dramatic increase in tidal volume delivery after endotracheal tube suctioning (downward deflections in PIP). The nurse had reported removal of a large amount of meconium from the airway at 0030 hours.

Reference: Chapter 17.